AF448809

THE KETOGENIC DIET WEIGHT LOSS

DR. FRANCIS GRACE

DISCLAIMER

Please note that this is a book and not drug for which it talks about and the information contained within this document is for entertainment and educational purposes only. All attempts have been made in other to provide up to date, reliable and accurate information. There is no warranties of any type is expressed or implied. Readers acknowledge that the author is by no means engaging in rendering of financial or legal, professional or medical advice. The content of this book has been derived from many sources. Please consult any licensed professional before attempting any step outlined in this book.

CONTENTS

TAPE ESTIMATIONS

MAKING CHANGES ACCORDING TO YOUR KETO DIET

CHAPTER EIGHTEEN

THE BEST PROCEDURE TO ADJUST TO ACTUATE KETOSIS

OBJECTIVES

Before the fruition of this guide, you'll have all that you have to begin the ketogenic diet to get logically fit the correct way — to the extent may be attainable.

CHAPTER ONE

INTRODUCTION

The ketogenic diet puts your body into a condition of ketosis, which over the long haul enables you to utilize fat for centrality.

Fat using is only a solitary of the different positive conditions of ketosis that overhauls all around flourishing and makes it a reasonable mechanical get together for weight decline.

Keto has a gathering following for an authentic diversion: it makes you feel impossible. Keto-ers feel consistently satisfied for the range of the day and have broadened vitality levels, both physical and mental, inciting:

- Fewer longings

- Lower caloric affirmation

- More impediment

- More physical action.

These great conditions all add to weight decline; regardless, keto isn't synonymous with weight decline.

A long way from being an appeal instrument, the ketogenic diet takes right and steady after and acclimation to work. You require a uniformity of the correct macros, rational target setting and following to take you closer to accomplishing your weight decline goals.

WHAT IS KETOSIS AND IN WHAT CAPACITY MAY IT ADVANCE FAT MISFORTUNE?

The ketogenic diet advances and deals with ketosis.

Ketosis is a metabolic state where your body uses fat as opposed to glucose from starches as its essential wellspring of essentialness.

To accomplish ketosis, you quit outfitting your body with carbs and sugar. This exhausts your set away glucose — for the most part called glycogen — and your glucose and insulin levels rot. Your body begins to filter for a substitute wellspring of fuel (fat), discharges it and copies it for noteworthiness.

Thusly, weight decline on keto.

In light of the reduction of glucose and growth in the absorption of fat, ketosis has a tremendous proportion of central focuses — its uncommon capacity to begin weight decline is only a solitary of them. Different individuals use ketosis as a treatment for epilepsy, diabetes and through and through disease.

Right when your body eats up fat, it produces ketones. Without ketones, you're not in ketosis. Along these lines, the ketogenic diet's sole reason behind existing is to help and impel ketone creation.

WHAT ARE KETONES?

Ketones are the metabolic fuel passed on when your body shifts into fat-using mode.

Glucose and ketones are the essential significance sources utilized by the cerebrum. Consider ketones the helper control wellspring of your body.

Going before the occurrence to development, when our precursors were searcher gatherers, they fasted once in a while. Precisely when sustenance was extraordinary, they didn't have a decision yet to trust that an obliging time will seek after for sustenance and cook it.

They had a low affirmation of carbs and protein and in this way were inadvertently running on ketones. Changing over set away fat into centrality is planned for our survival and a trademark bit of human closeness.

Your body uses fat to utilize and pass on ketones at whatever point glucose sources are low or drained, for example,

- during fasting

- after conceded work out

- when you eat a ketogenic diet.

Lipase (a force in charge of fat breakdown) discharges set away triglycerides (fats). These unsaturated fats go to your liver and your liver changes them into ketones.

There are three sorts of ketone bodies:

- Acetoacetate – amidst the breakdown of long-and medium-chain unsaturated fats for centrality, acetoacetate is passed on first.

- Acetone – Quickly, CH3)2CO is in like way passed on as a side effect of acetoacetate.

Both of these ketone bodies, when not utilized, spill into your pee and breath, making pee and breath testing a promising estimation of paying little personality to whether you're going into ketosis. More on this underneath in How to Test Ketone Levels.

•   Beta-hydroxybutyrate (BHB) – Not by any stretch of the imagination a ketone however rather a particle. Its main work in the ketogenic diet exploits it as the fundamental ketone body. BHB is composed by your liver from acetoacetate. BHB is fundamental in light of the manner in which that it can uninhibitedly skim all through your body in your blood, crossing different tissues where unmistakable atoms can't. It enters the mitochondria and gets changed into ATP (adenosine triphosphate), the importance cash of your cells. BHB = ATP = significance!

Since you comprehend what ketones are and how ketosis limits, you no doubt need to know why you ought to consider eating a ketogenic diet — the eating plan that advances ketosis.

CHAPTER TWO

THE UPSIDES OF KETOSIS

The upsides of ketones start from your body using fat for fuel and the chop down glucose and insulin in your blood.

The upsides of ketosis include:

• Body fat using

• Mental clearness and broadened keenness

• Improved physical vitality

• No feeling of hardship since you experience less yearning

• Steady glucose levels from in every way that really matters no affirmation of refined carbs

• Skin overhauls in those with skin break out

- Improved triglyceride and cholesterol levels

- Hormone control — ladies who go on keto report less authentic responses of PMS.

Near the accommodating inclinations of ketones, different individuals begin to look all starry looked toward at keto in light of the manner by which it makes them feel both soundly and physically.

Suggested Looking at

- The Most conspicuous Ketogenic Diet Central focuses

- Is Ketosis Safe?

- What Are Ketones?

- Perfect Keto Clients Guide

- How to Deal with Ketosis

- When and How to Improve With Ketones

- Why Supplement With Exogenous Ketones?

- The Specific Sorts of Ketone Upgrades

- What is AcetoAcetate?

- What is Beta-HydroxyButyrate (BHB)?

- What is CH3)2CO?

- Perfect Keto Ketone Testing Strips

CHAPTER THREE

THE KETOGENIC DIET WEIGHT DIMINISHING OUTCOMES

The ketogenic diet is an appropriate instrument for weight decline in context of the energizing reduction in carb attestation, driving your body to eat up fat rather than carbs for vitality.

Results move among people by virtue of two or three factors, for example, insulin limitation and momentous body creation. In any case, keto has reliably lead to a decrease in weight and muscle to fat extent in a wide degree of conditions including yet not constrained to stoutness, type 2 diabetes and athletic execution.

A randomized control examine in 2017 separated the effects of a ketogenic diet united with Crossfit preparing on body sythesis and execution. Results from this examination expected that subjects following a low-starch ketogenic diet (LCKD) completely diminished body weight, muscle to fat extent and fat mass showed up diversely in connection to those in the control gathering.

The subjects following the ketogenic diet:

1.   Lost a run of the mill of 3.45 kilograms (7.6 pounds) showed up contrastingly in connection to those in the control accumulate who had no mishap in body weight.

2.   Lost a run of the mill of 2.6% muscle to fat extent while those in the control gather did not lose anyone fat.

3.   Lost all around 2.83 kilograms (6.2 pounds) of fat mass (the bit of the body made through and through out of fat) showed up contrastingly in connection to the control assemble who did not lose any fat mass.

4.   Maintained fit burden to vague degree from those in the control gathering.

5.   Improved Crossfit execution to undefined degree from those in the control gathering.

Dashti et al. played out an examination in 2004 viewing the entire arrangement effects of a ketogenic diet in fat patients and found the accompanying:

1.   The weight and weight archive of the patients decreased essentially.

2.   The component of absolute cholesterol decreased from week 1 to week 24.

1.   HDL cholesterol (the unimaginable one) levels on an essential dimension expanded.

2.   LDL cholesterol (the terrible one) levels on an extremely essential dimension reduced after treatment.

3.   The segment of triglycerides (fat) decreased on an essential dimension following 24 weeks of treatment.

4.   The segment of blood glucose basically diminished.

Partsalaki et al. completed an examination in 2012 looking effects of a ketogenic diet versus a hypocaloric diet in overwhelming kids and adolescents. Results showed up:

•   Children following the ketogenic diet fundamentally lessened body weight, fat mass, midsection breaking point and fasting insulin levels.

•   The kids in the ketogenic diet bunch in a general sense reduced a marker of insulin obstruction known as homeostatic model examination insulin impediment (HOMA-IR) to a more unquestionable degree than those following a hypocaloric diet.

- An fundamental marker of insulin affectability and cardiovascular disease — known as high atomic weight (HMW) adiponectin — unmitigated stretched out in the ketogenic diet gathering at any rate not in the hypocaloric diet gathering.

Similarly, a continuous report looking effects of a low-starch ketogenic diet versus a low-glycemic record diet in sort 2 diabetics was driven.

Results from this examination expected that people following the ketogenic diet had in a general sense progressively basic updates in weight decline, hemoglobin A1c, and high thickness lipoprotein (HDL) cholesterol showed up distinctively in connection to the low-glycemic record diet gathering:

Those following a ketogenic diet:

1. Lost everything considered 11.1 kilograms (24.5 pounds) emerged from those

following the low-glycemic record diet who lost all around 6.9 kilograms (15.2 pounds)

2.   Reduced their HbA1c levels by 1.5% veered from the low-glycemic rundown diet complete who essentially reduced their HbA1c levels by 0.5%.

3.   Increased their HDL cholesterol everything contemplated 5.6 mg/dL showed up diversely in connection to those in the low-glycemic rundown store up who had no enlargements in HDL cholesterol.

4.   Diabetes cures were decreased or disposed of in 95.2% of people in the ketogenic diet collect versus just 62% of people in the low-glycemic record gathering.

The ketogenic diet works for weight decline since it's based around high fat, elegant protein and low carb usage.

Regardless, I Thought Fat Was Horrendous For You?

There's a normal misguided judgment that fat is awful for you; regardless, this chaos neglects to acceptably address sound fats which are truth be told bravo.

Near other probably shown focal points, doused fats like medium-chain triglycerides (MCTs) go expressly to your liver to be utilized for importance.

The ketogenic diet, with its irregular condition of good fats, prompts a fat-adaptable metabolic state.

Fat-adjustment happens when your body winds up being continuously reasonable at eating up fat for fuel. The more you keep up a fat-versatile express, the more ketones you make.

The objective of a ketogenic diet is to keep up high extents of ketones so you can get the vast majority of the prizes that happen from being in ketosis.

A high fat, ketogenic diet is comparatively protein-saving: your body continues consuming fat and doesn't swing to protein as a vitality source.

The total Protein Can I Really Eat?

Protein is essential on keto as well. In a perfect world, you should debilitate 0.8 grams of protein per pound of slight weight. This will dismiss muscle hardship.

To enroll your thin weight, you need to:

•   Calculate your muscle versus fat extent. Snap here to investigate how.

•   Subtract your muscle versus fat % from 100%. This will be your meager weight %.

- Multiply your fit weight % by your all out weight.

Concentrated on that 0.8 grams per pound of fit weight is an excessive amount of protein?

Truly on a keto diet, you can eat considerably more protein than the standard 10-15% of all out calories (that some remarkable sources advance) without being kicked out of ketosis.

An excess of protein won't raise your blood glucose and decline your ketone levels. That is only a fantasy.

Low-Carb Isn't Ketogenic

The separation among ketogenic and low-carb stays away from sustenance is that the ketogenic diet goes for ketosis.

Other low-carb eats less most likely won't have a sufficiently colossal decline in carb admission to move your osmosis into making and eating up ketones for fuel.

Notwithstanding, express sorts of keto counts calories do cause them to breathe in space with carb and protein use.

The 4 Sorts of Ketogenic Diets

Like sporadic fasting, you can change the ketogenic diet as shown by your goals or necessities.

There are four normal sorts of ketogenic counts calories:

•   The Standard Ketogenic Diet (SKD): Most normal and proposed rendition of the diet:20-50 grams of net carbs reliably, moderate protein affirmation and high fat insistence.

•   Targeted Ketogenic Diet (TKD): "Facilitated" for vitality around your exercises: 25-50 grams of net carbs or less around 30 minutes to an hour going before work out

- Cyclical Ketogenic Diet (CKD): Like irregular fasting "Down Day Up Day" or the 5/2 cycle, CKD fuses eating a low-carb, ketogenic diet for two or three days looked for after by a couple of long stretches of eating high-carb.

- High-Protein Ketogenic Diet: The SKD exchanged with extra extents of protein that could be perfect for constantly first rate contenders

CHAPTER FOUR

WHAT TO GOBBLE AND WHAT TO KEEP UP A KEY DIVISION FROM ON THE KETO DIET

Ketogenic sustenances are mind blowing, entire, trademark sustenances dealt with as little as could be typical the circumstance being what it is. To keep up a key partition from organized sustenances, different keto-ers need to make everything themselves, from burgers to hand created ghee).

Ketogenic sustenances are high in fat, pleasing in protein and obviously, low carb.

The most extraordinary discovers a ketogenic diet merge not seeing the quality and structure of your sustenance and being careless about your carb usage.

To get increasingly slim on keto you should:

•	Count carbs — even shrouded carbs found in flavors, vegetables and beverages.

•	Watch your sugar grant: this fuses sugars, consequences of the earth happening sugars in dairy. On the off chance that you should utilize a sugar, stay with stevia or pick other keto-obliging sugars.

•	Watch your calories. Attempt not to beat your calorie spending plan. To get alive and well you have to eat not as much as what you use. All figurings and estimations are talked about underneath.

•	Be aware of your sustenance when all is said in done. Keep up a key detachment from managed sustenance. Despite how low-carb or "keto" it might be, if it's flooding with garbage you're in an ideal condition maintaining a strategic distance from it.

•	Drink a lot of water. Carbs are praised for holding water, so keto's low-carb degree can incite snappier nonappearance of hydration and discouraging. Repay with water and keto-obliging beverages.

• Try discontinuous fasting to keep away from late night overabundances and enliven your ketone creation and weight decline.

Your carb and protein affirmation makes (or breaks) your ketogenic diet. You can change your macros as exhibited by what works for you, in any case the general macronutrient reaches are:

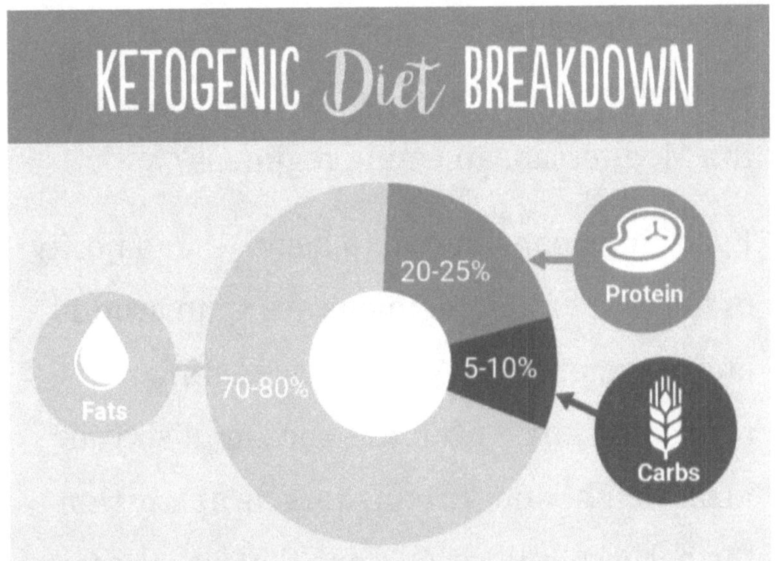

These can move as exhibited by your objectives, needs and body sythesis. Sorting out your ketogenic diet joins enrolling your macros.

Keto versus Unquestionably comprehended Weight decline Diets: Atkins, Paleo, Mediterranean

Keto has been requested "Atkins on steroids" and is once in a while emerged from different eating regimens like paleo and the Mediterranean eating plan. What are the practically identical characteristics and separations between keto, Atkins, paleo and the Mediterranean eating regimens?

Everything considered, to begin, the majority of the four eating regimens are spun around entire sustenance. Any of these eating regimens can be utilized to accomplish your ideal weight and thriving targets at any rate the basic complexities come down to the far reaching scale transports and unmistakably, ketosis.

CHAPTER FIVE

KETO AND ATKINS

The Atkins diet, formally called the Atkins Solid Rationality, was developed by methods for cardiologist Dr. Robert Atkins as a heap decline device subject to "eating right, not less."

The similarities: Both the ketogenic and Atkins consumes less calories diminish your insistence of carbs and sugar while pushing you toward eating entire, solid sustenances.

At whatever point done correctly, the outcome is ketosis, weight abatement and better mental sharpness and physical vitality from the consistent fuel of ketones.

The capability: Atkins has four stages. The affirmation and altering stages (Stage 1 and 2) take after the ketogenic diet generally nearly.

- Phase 1 (Determination) merges gobbling up low carbs at 20-25 grams of net carbs reliably. After choice, you well ordered reintroduce and increment your carb license once again, until the minute that you locate the ideal total that fulfills you without understanding extra weight gain.

- Phase 2 (Modifying) has 25-50 grams net carbs reliably.

- Phase 3 (Modifying or pre-support) has 50-80 grams net carbs reliably.

- Phase 4 (Backing) has 80-100 grams of net carb grant well ordered.

In the ketogenic diet, the carb, protein and fat macros are reinforced in their distributed bits to influence and keep up a condition of ketosis.

The Managers of Atkins:

- Can be more clear to keep up than keto, particularly for individuals who experience issues keeping up a key partition from carbs.

- Ideal for tenderfoots to encounter ketosis and the majority of the inclinations in the principal stages while endeavoring assorted things with various factors and after that keeping up ketosis in the event that they decide to.

KETO AND PALEO

The paleo or paleolithic eating routine — besides called the mountain man diet, searcher gatherer diet or Stone Age diet — depends after utilizing the sustenances accessible to our predecessors in their searcher gatherer days and the beginning of agriculture,about 10,000 years sooner.

With paleo, organized sustenance is out. This surmises no sugar or flour-based sustenances since passing on sugar and getting ready wheat wasn't organized yet in those days.

Anything you could seek after, catch, pick or passage starting from the most dependable stage is in, for example, meat, point, common things, nuts and vegetables.

The practically identical characteristics: Both the ketogenic and paleo eats less are rich in non-dull vegetables. Both in like way confine sugar, grains, vegetables and suggest incredible creature proteins and fats.

The refinements:

For whatever time range that your gut doesn't have an issue disconnecting them, keto is significantly alright with full-fat, all essential dairy — cheddar, margarine, ghee. Then again, paleo keeps away from whatever can trade off the gut like dairy.

Emerged from the express low carb obstruction of the ketogenic diet, paleo does not continue depleting vegetables and sugary standard things, making it close difficult to get into ketosis.

The Specialists of Paleo:

- Can be perfect for wellbeing buffs who perform well ordered, high-control works out.

- Good for veggie sweethearts and vegetarians.

CHAPTER SIX

KETO AND THE MEDITERRANEAN EATING CALENDAR

Physiologist Dr. Ancel Keys saw that the Mediterranean individuals living in southern Europe (Greece, Italy, Crete) had much lower dangers of coronary disorder than Americans. He recorded what they ate and the Mediterranean eating routine was considered. This eating routine contains generally of fish, vegetables, trademark things, seeds, beans, olive oil, nuts, cheddar, yogurt and grains. Poultry and eggs eaten each two days, red meat kept to 3 ounces for reliably and a glass or two of wine well ordered.

The tantamount characteristics: Like keto, the Mediterranean eating routine supplements clear, entire sustenances.

The refinements: The Mediterranean eating routine is ordinarily low-fat, with non-ketogenic net carbs starting from grains like bread, quinoa, diminish tinted rice, dull aftereffects of the soil.

The Stars of the Mediterranean Eating routine:

- The most clear of the four weight control plans depicted here
- Avoids extraordinarily arranged sustenances like paleo.

The Takeaway

The ketogenic diet has one reason: to affect ketosis, devouring fat as opposed to carbs. Exchange eating regimens have their a great deal of medicinal points of interest, particularly the Mediterranean eating routine, and all of them help with weight decrease, anyway simply the ketogenic diet causes you affect and care for ketosis.

The point of convergence of these weight control plans is to eat healthy, whole sustenances that are as close nature as could sensibly be normal. To be sure, even without the exhaustive after required on keto, in spite of all that you have to watch the proportion of sustenance you are consuming on these eating regimens in order to accomplish the favorable circumstances.

Keto is presently considered "Atkins on steroids." on the off chance that you're restless to get the benefits of being in ketosis, the paleo and Mediterranean weight control plans can be versatile to activate a ketogenic state. Simply displace most of the bread and tasteless root vegetables with more oil, oily meats and fish and low-carb nuts.

We incorporate every one of the three of the above weight control anticipates Perfect Keto:

- Comparing Keto versus the Mediterranean Eating routine
- The Ketogenic Diet versus the Atkins Diet
- Paleo versus Ketogenic Diet

Organizing a Keto Plan for Weight decrease

Using the ketogenic diet for weight decrease is connected to following and registering:

- Macros
- Ketone levels
- Stress
- Exercise yield
- Sleep

Anything out of equality — like too much protein or over the top exercise — can achieve something as fundamental as moderate your headway into ketosis, or something continuously grave like aggravate your prosperity.

Your very own needs and targets choose a ton when using the ketogenic diet for weight decrease. The most basic development is registering (and clinging to) your macros.

Using a Keto Full-scale Analyst

To register your macros, start with a huge scale analyst (Understanding: we have one you can use in vain).

In case you use a wellbeing application like MyFitnessPal, you've formally used an enormous scale smaller than expected PC, in spite of the way that the free type of the application just gives you a calorie spending plan.

In figuring your macros, you choose your confirmation of carbs, protein and fat according to your BMR (basal metabolic rate), development level, body sythesis and weight decrease targets.

Processing your macros is key to achieving your destinations.

So what goes into registering your macros?

1: Your Basal Metabolic Rate (BMR)

Your BMR is the base number of calories you need to support your body's essential limits (breathing, heart throbbing, preparing sustenance) without checking the calories required for step by step activities and exercise.

Your age, sexual introduction, stature and weight pick your BMR.

- Weight and stature: The more significant you are, the more calories you require so your organs can bolster you.

- Age: Mass goes down as you age, which can decrease your BMR.

- Gender: Body game-plan contrasts among people.

We get a near to figuring of BMR utilizing the Harris-Benedict condition:

- BMR condition for men = 66 + (6.2 x Burden in pounds) + (12.7 x Stature in inches) − (6.76 x Age)

- BMR condition for ladies = 655.1 + (4.35 x Burden in pounds) + (4.7 x Stature in inches) – (4.7 x Age)

For instance:

A 28-year old individual gauging 130 pounds and remaining at 5'2 would discover her BMR as:

- 665.1 + 565.1 + 291.4 – 131.6 = 1390 calories expected to support huge point of confinement

A 28-year more established individual gauging 182 pounds and remaining at 6'1 would figure his BMR as:

- 66 + 1128.4 + 914.4 – 189.28 = 1919.52 calories expected to support veritable farthest point

2: Your All out Every day Criticalness Use (TDEE)

Your TDEE unites a wide extent of activity, paying little notice to whether it's your reliably practice or physically requesting days at work or at home. This issues in enrolling your calories and macros.

Utilize these numbers as a guide:

- 1.2: Beside zero exercise

- 1.375: Light exercise, 1-3 days out of reliably

- 1.55: Moderate exercise, 3-5 days out of reliably

- 1.725: Hard exercise, 6-7 days out of reliably

- 1.9: Particularly certifiable exercise

Which number best matches your action level? Augmentation that number by the BMR number you chose previously. The thing is your complete well-ordered calorie use, or all out calorie eat up.

For instance, a lady with a BMR of 1500 who conservatives exercise would have this equation: 1500 x 1.55 to get her all out well ordered calorie use, 2,325.

She exhausts 2,325 calories to support her body and reliably works out.

3: Your Body Game-plan: Muscle versus fat extent and Fit Weight

Your muscle versus fat extent picks your fit weight — the all out pile of your body less your fat mass — which along these lines picks the extent of protein you have to keep up your muscles.

This is the reason most rec focuses have skinfold calipers, which are incredibly close right. You can buy a couple on the web.

Assorted approaches to manage assess muscle to fat extent are:

• DEXA check. This addresses twofold vitality x-column absorptiometry, measures bone mineral thickness, at any rate can in like way completely measure your muscle versus fat extent. It's expensive and can take as long as 30 minutes, in any case it is the best quality measurement for assessing muscle to fat extent.

• Body estimations. Applications and online instruments give muscle versus fat counts utilizing your stature, weight and the tape estimations of your neck, mid-district, and hips.

• Photos. Visual evaluations give a more careful check than body estimations. Take a full body photograph of yourself and a brief timeframe later separation it and the photographs of various individuals. Continue taking photographs. It will end up being useful later as you screen your headway.

4: Discovering Your Muscle versus fat and Slender Weight

Subtract your muscle to fat extent from your weight and you get your fit weight.

Convert your muscle to fat extent into pounds first. For instance, your muscle versus fat is 25% and you gauge 150 pounds.

150 pounds x .25 = 37.5 pounds of muscle to fat extent.

Next, subtract that from your weight.

150 pounds − 37.5 pounds of fat = 112.5 pounds of thin weight.

Spare your number. You'll utilize it later to decide your protein.

5: Your Weight decline Objectives

To accomplish weight decline, your absolute calorie license every day should be in a need:

you eat up less calories than your all out well ordered use.

A 10%-20% lack, or even 30% in the event that you can oversee, is a traditional range. Basically don't go over a 30% decay every day since it can cause entire arrangement issues.

For instance, to diminish by 20%, duplicate your all out calorie usage by 0.20. Subtract that total from your all out calorie use.

That is your all out well ordered calories, the most over the top extent of calories you ought to expend every day. Eating not as much as what you eat up well ordered would exhaust off the store you need to lose.

HANDLING YOUR CARBS

On the ketogenic diet, sugars make up 5%-10% of complete calories everything considered.

For a huge number people, that is around 20-50 net grams for reliably.

Recipe: (mean calorie use x % of calories from carbs)/4

Duplicate your complete calories by the element of carbs and section it by 4 to get grams.

For an all out every day calorie assertion of 2000 with the ketogenic 5% to 10% carbs, the equation would be:

2000 x 0.05 or 0.10 = 100 to 200 calories from carbs

200/4 = 25g to 50g of carbs reliably.

CHAPTER SEVEN

FINDING YOUR PROTEIN

On the ketogenic diet, your protein certification ought to be moderate at about 20% to 25% of your complete calories, enough to deal with muscle, in any case not all that much that it impacts ketosis.

Your protein insistence should bolster your improvement level and keep up your slight weight, which you chose previously.

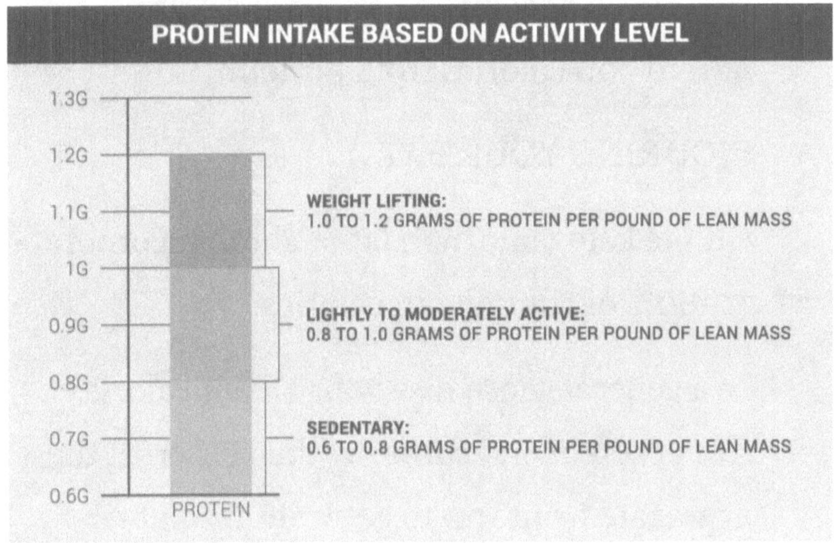

Utilize these degrees to pick your ideal protein use. Begin with the lower grams number.

For instance, a pleasantly incredible female gauging 150 pounds and has 112.5 pounds of thin weight will require 90-112.5 grams of protein reliably. Addition that by 4 to enlist 360-450 calories from protein for reliably.

Next, duplicate your all out calories by 0.20 to 0.25 to ensure your protein from calories fit inside that rate.

E.g., 2000 absolute calories x 0.20 or 0.25 = 400 to 500 calories from protein.

FIGURING YOUR FAT

On the ketogenic diet, fat ought to incorporate 70-80% of your all out calories.

In a general sense fuse your all out calories from protein and carbs, by then subtract the aggregate from 100 to get your absolute calories of fat.

100 to 200 calories of carbs + 400 to 500 calories of protein = 500 to 700 calories

2000 all out calories − 500 to 700 = 1500 to 1300 calories from fat

Fat has 9 calories for each gram so we separate the calories by 9 to get grams. 1500 or 1300/9 = 167g or 144g of fat.

The above methods your carbs, protein and fat macros give you a range to work in, not ensured right and accurate, yet rather you can change. Your body will uncover to you what it needs and what it increases in value. Some keto-ers report remaining in ketosis in fluctuating extents of carbs and protein.

CHAPTER EIGHT

PRACTICING ON THE KETO DIET

The astounding state of eating less and practicing more to get logically fit is obsolete, false and unsustainable.

What you eat matters, and the ketogenic diet is one of the contraptions for weight decline where this is most recognizably plainly obvious.

Exercise advances thin muscle building, progressively basic bone quality and improved stamina and resolute quality. Exercise in like way encounters your glycogen stores, helping you get into ketosis snappier. So consider practice to be device to accomplish these focal points as opposed to just to shed pounds.

4 Sorts of Development In Ketosis

•   Aerobic works out: Cardio. Props up more than three minutes to raise your pulse.

Lower compel, solid state cardio is fat eating up, making it inviting for the keto prosperity sustenance nut.

•	Anaerobic works out: HIIT or weight wanting to assemble muscle. Over the top, short effects of centrality to drive quality and speed. Sugars are the fundamental fuel for anaerobic exercise, so fat alone can't give enough vitality to this kind of movement.

•	Flexibility works out: Yoga and stretches, for overhauling muscle and joint improvement, and keeping wounds from the shortening of muscles after some time.

•	Stability works out: Center preparing, Pilates, balance works out, yoga. Improves game-plan, balance, muscle quality and headway control.

When you're in ketosis, the movement control matters:

• During low-drive oxygen consuming development, the body uses fat as its principal vitality source.

- During high-control oxygen exhausting activity, starches are normally the basic criticalness source.

This is the reason you consider your action level while figuring your macros. When you begin the ketogenic diet, the SKD (standard ketogenic diet) may not be sufficient to fuel your exercises.

Utilize the focused on ketogenic diet (TKD).

CHAPTER NINE

FACILITATED KETOGENIC DIET AND FAT CHANGE

In the TKD, you eat 15 to 30 grams of quick acting carbs, similar to normal thing, inside 30 minutes before your movement or potentially inside 30 minutes after your action.

This outfits your muscles with the best extent of glycogen to perform amidst arranging and recuperate some time later. The carbs you fumes are utilized unmistakably along these lines and keep the danger of getting kicked out of ketosis.

Fortunately the more you remain in ketosis, the more your body ends up fat-versatile and legitimately able at using fat for vitality, a trademark technique that your body winds up languid at when reliably outfitted with carbs.

FOCAL POINTS OF PRACTICING WHILE IN KETOSIS

A long way from frustrating exercises, ketosis adds central focuses to practice that update its assistance for when in doubt wellbeing and weight decline.

In one examination, showed up contrastingly in connection to the general population who ate a high-carb diet, ultra-consistency contenders who ate a low-carb diet for a common of 20 months ate up 2-3 times powerfully fat amidst a three-hour-long run.

In a near report, the low-carb aggregate utilized and reestablished vague extent of muscle glycogen from the high-carb gathering.

Being in ketosis may in like way help imagine weakness amidst longer events of oxygen eating up activity. Likewise, ketosis has been appeared to help with blood glucose upkeep amidst action in vigorous people.

As referenced over, the power of keto-adjustment helps low-carb weight watchers perform better in a wide scope of activity with less carbs after some time.

Swear off overtraining. Overtraining raises your cortisol levels. Cortisol, the weight hormone, impacts your body to acknowledge you're in battle or flight mode, raising your insulin and glucose, not something you require on keto.

SPORADIC FASTING WITH THE KETO DIET

Sporadic fasting is regularly done related to the ketogenic diet. The two techniques help one another. Fasting causes you get into ketosis, and ketosis invigorates you smart even more effectively.

Together, they eat up a gigantic measure of fat and may enable you to get progressively fit snappier. Investigate our guide on

Discontinuous Fasting for more data on the most fit strategy to utilize erratic fasting with the ketogenic diet.

CHAPTER TEN

UTILIZING EXOGENOUS KETONES TO MOVE WEIGHT REDUCTION ON KETO

Exogenous ketones are ketone supplements that help your endogenous (inside) ketone creation and in the meantime give you minute importance when you require it.

They enable your body to enter ketosis by setting you up with ketones, urging your body to change to that noteworthiness source rather than glucose. They put you on an anticipated fat eat up and give you vitality to exhaust work out.

Exogenous ketones are a notable gadget for weight decline since they help you with exercises and amidst fasting, give you an immaculate stun of imperativeness and completion you off with ketones, are incomprehensible for exercise execution and fulfill your aching without breaking your quick.

You may have heard somebody state they need to urge down ketones since they taste appalling. We explain why they frequently do, and that is an expansive piece of why Faultless Keto was developed: to make ketones sensibly available (i.e., wonderful) to everybody.

To plot, at present Faultless Keto Base comes in Chocolate, Peaches and Cream, Vanilla and Espresso flavors. Impeccable Keto Perform Pre-Exercise arrives in a reviving lemon update.

To utilize ketones for fat eating up:

Take one scoop of Immaculate Keto Base at whatever point in the midst of meals for predictable fat eating up.

To utilize ketones to get into ketosis (or get over into it following a cheat day):

Take ½ a scoop of Immaculate Keto Base at whatever point you need to get into ketosis rapidly similarly as direct after a supper that is heavier on starches than foreseen.

To utilize ketones for criticalness amidst the keto headway or fasting:

Before an action that will be 45 minutes or more, take a full scoop. By then take another ½ of a scoop for dependably surpassing two critical bunches of unending work you do. You can take either Consummate Keto Base or Immaculate Keto Perform Pre-work out. Note that it's not encouraged to do considerable exercises while changing to keto or amidst your quick.

CHAPTER ELEVEN

UTILIZING ASSORTED ENHANCEMENTS FOR A KETOGENIC DIET

• Minerals/Electrolytes: Getting a handle on a ketogenic diet will change the manner by which your body uses (and loses) certain minerals. Not supplanting these minerals can prompt signs of the "keto influenza, for example, wooziness, cerebral pains, check, muscle fits and fatigue. Recommend this article for tips on the most fit system to abrogate standard minerals, for example, sodium, potassium, magnesium and calcium.

• Fish Oil

☐ Fish oil is a surprising wellspring of omega 3s and a trademark adversary of incendiary. Eating up around 3000-5000 mg of fish oil every day with high EPA/DHA is proposed. One top notch source is Antarctic Krill Oil. Assurance that whichever source you pick, it has the IFOS five star rating and is wandered with a FOS support.

- MCT Powder

☐ MCT oil powder is a charming sort of dietary fat promptly eaten up by the body and has a wide degree of helpful focal points. Supplementation with MCT powder can enable battle to depletion, cover craving, update thermogenesis (likewise called 'fat consuming') and help your body change as per utilizing ketones for fuel. A constant reliable audit displayed that MCTs can sensibly diminish body weight, mean muscle to fat extent, hip fringe, midsection edges, imply subcutaneous fat and regular fat. Look at this article for more data on the best way to deal with improve with MCTs.

- Collagen

☐ Collagen is a kind of protein that has been appeared to cover hunger, give realization emerged from different proteins like whey, casein, or soy, empower hold to bulk and even assistance to reduce the closeness of cellulite because of it's capacity to redesign skin versatility and thickness. Recommend this article for more data on the advantages of collagen and the most ideal approach to manage overhaul it in your eating schedule.

- Greens Powder

☐ Getting satisfactory extents of enhancements is essential to help sound weight decline and standard speaking thriving. Taking a multivitamin with manufactured fixings has been appeared, apparently, to be insufficient and a hard and fast maltreatment of cash. On the other hand, gobbling up a stunning greens powder conveyed using genuine, nutritious entire sustenances well-to-do in enhancements, minerals, cell strongholds, fiber and phytonutrients is an incredibly upgraded approach to manage streamline thriving and future. See this article for more data on improving with a high measure, persuading greens powder.

•   Probiotics

☐   Gut thriving is fundamental for anybody needing to get progressively fit and expansion when all is said in done wellbeing. It isn't exceptional for the general population who move to a ketogenic diet to have an adjustment in the period of minute life frames in their colon (paying little mind to the way that less an unpleasant thing – only a change). To help bolster this change and growth the solid little animals in your gut, take a stab at eating up logically created sustenances, for example, sauerkraut, kimchi or kefir or possibly supplement with a top of the line probiotic.

- Vitamin D

☐ It's assessed that over part of individuals are lacking in Enhancement D around the world. Despite the manner in which that Supplement D doesn't acknowledge a significant movement in paying little personality to whether you are in ketosis, it is in charge of controlling obstacle, exacerbation, hormones and assisting with electrolyte ingestion — all parts fundamental for weight decline and all around flourishing. Also, mulls over assistance the speedy focal points of enhancement D for weight reduction. You can check your Enhancement D levels with a reasonable blood test and after that supplement as necessities be. While redesigning, pick Supplement D3 as the shape's best eaten up by your body.

- L-Glutamine

☐ L-glutamine is an amino damaging with different points of confinement in your body including going about as a weighty cancer prevention agent. Research demonstrates that L-glutamine can empower evening out to out blood glucose levels and has been embraced to help diminish sugar longings. Redesigning with L-glutamine (about ½-1 teaspoon powdered packaging or 500 mg isolate) may help in reducing carb/sugar longings and help in your ketogenic weight decline experience.

- Ox Bile

o Those who've had their gallbladder removed may require bull bile supplementation to help their body in segregating fats and help in when in doubt assimilation. Right when taken with an eat up, bull bile gives a concentrated wellspring of bile which replaces the bile that would have been discharged by your gallbladder. As referenced officially, bona fide dealing with is essential to helping help in weight decline and improving all around flourishing and prosperity.

CHAPTER TWELVE

SUPERVISING WEIGHT REDUCTION LEVELS ON THE KETOGENIC DIET

Keto-ers get a kick out of the smart progress they see with the ketogenic diet. There's reliably an energetic drop in burden as you lose those carbs and water weight.

The measurement comes straightaway: your weight abatement backs way off or even appears to stop as you begin losing genuine fat. You can't move beyond it paying little regard to how hard you try.

A couple of basic center interests:

- 1 to 2 pounds seven days is sound weight decline. You may lose progressively, yet paying little heed to all that you're getting increasingly slim. Not losing anything for seven days from time to time is alright.

- Plateaus happen intentionally. Inspect your measurement so you can settle it.

INVESTIGATING YOUR MEASUREMENT

At whatever point you quit getting dynamically fit, check whether any of the going with could be the reasons and complete the basic changes.

FACTORS THAT AFFECT WEIGHT LOSS ON KETO

EATING TOO MANY CARBS

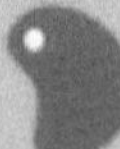

EATING TOO MUCH PROTEIN

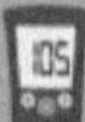

NOT TRACKING KETONE LEVELS OFTEN

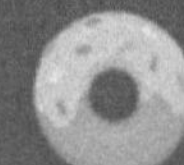

EATING TOO MANY CALORIES

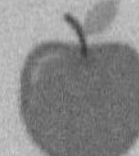

NOT BEING MINDFUL OF
TYPES OF KETO FOODS

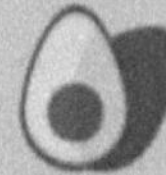

NOT EATING REAL WHOLE FOODS

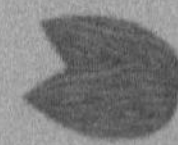

EATING TOO MANY NUTS

NOT INCORPORATING FASTING

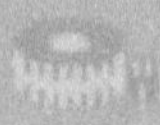

GETTING CLOSER TO YOUR GOAL WEIGHT

NOT GETTING ENOUGH SLEEP

BEING STRESSED OUT

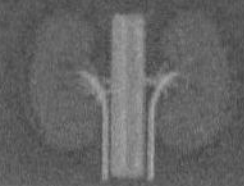

ADRENAL OR THYROID CONCERNS

- Probiotics

☐ Gut thriving is fundamental for anybody needing to get progressively fit and expansion when all is said in done wellbeing. It isn't exceptional for the general population who move to a ketogenic diet to have an adjustment in the period of minute life frames in their colon (paying little mind to the way that less an unpleasant thing – only a change). To help bolster this change and growth the solid little animals in your gut, take a stab at eating up logically created sustenances, for example, sauerkraut, kimchi or kefir or possibly supplement with a top of the line probiotic.

- Vitamin D

☐ It's assessed that over part of individuals are lacking in Enhancement D around the world. Despite the manner in which that Supplement D doesn't acknowledge a significant movement in paying little personality to whether you are in ketosis, it is in charge of controlling obstacle, exacerbation, hormones and assisting with electrolyte ingestion — all parts fundamental for weight decline and all around flourishing. Also, mulls over assistance the speedy focal points of enhancement D for weight reduction. You can check your Enhancement D levels with a reasonable blood test and after that supplement as necessities be. While redesigning, pick Supplement D3 as the shape's best eaten up by your body.

- L-Glutamine

☐ L-glutamine is an amino damaging with different points of confinement in your body including going about as a weighty cancer prevention agent. Research demonstrates that L-glutamine can empower evening out to out blood glucose levels and has been embraced to help diminish sugar longings. Redesigning with L-glutamine (about ½-1 teaspoon powdered packaging or 500 mg isolate) may help in reducing carb/sugar longings and help in your ketogenic weight decline experience.

- Ox Bile

o	Those who've had their gallbladder removed may require bull bile supplementation to help their body in segregating fats and help in when in doubt assimilation. Right when taken with an eat up, bull bile gives a concentrated wellspring of bile which replaces the bile that would have been discharged by your gallbladder. As referenced officially, bona fide dealing with is essential to helping help in weight decline and improving all around flourishing and prosperity.

CHAPTER THIRTEEN

SUPERVISING WEIGHT REDUCTION
LEVELS ON THE KETOGENIC DIET

Keto-ers get a kick out of the smart progress
they see with the ketogenic diet. There's
reliably an energetic drop in burden as you
lose those carbs and water weight.

The measurement comes straightaway: your
weight abatement backs way off or even
appears to stop as you begin losing genuine
fat. You can't move beyond it paying little
regard to how hard you try.

A couple of basic center interests:

•	1 to 2 pounds seven days is sound weight
decline. You may lose progressively, yet
paying little heed to all that you're getting
increasingly slim. Not losing anything for
seven days from time to time is alright.

- Plateaus happen intentionally. Inspect your measurement so you can settle it.

INVESTIGATING YOUR MEASUREMENT

At whatever point you quit getting dynamically fit, check whether any of the going with could be the reasons and complete the basic changes.

CHECKING KETONE LEVELS BY RESPONSES

When you're new out of testing gear, the going with signs can demonstrate your movement or condition of ketosis.

You should at present utilize the above gadgets to quantify your ketones, yet these signs can tell you're progressing agreeably, in any event.

Expanded Thirst, Dry Tissues: On the ketogenic diet, your body will encounter abundance glycogen and will manufacture the extent of pee. You're also losing the water-bolster some bit of carb affirmation. Repay with water and electrolytes.

Mental Lucidity and Better Gratefulness: Your cerebrum reliably uses a lot of essentialness. On carbs, the variances in your insulin levels can cause hugeness swings. In ketosis, your mind will utilize an irrefutably obvious wellspring of fuel: ketones from your fat stores or your updates, acknowledging better efficiency and mental execution.

Less Yearning and Needs: When your body ends up used to utilizing ketones, you will start utilizing fat to seclude into ketones to use for essentialness. Since your body has such a steady supply of vitality, it doesn't pine for sustenance the manner by which it did when your importance was subject to starch affirmation.

Powerfully Continued with Centrality: 90-120 minutes after you eat sugars, your body doesn't have promptly accessible vitality passed on from the mitochondria in your phones, so you begin "squashing" or chopping down your vitality. When you are in ketosis, your body can keep running off your muscle versus fat, which is an on a very basic level boundless wellspring of fuel. This keeps any sort of incident.

Not Breath: CH3)2CO levels in the breath under solid ketosis ought not be satisfactorily high to cause a perceptible fragrance.

One customary deluding we've been made mindful of is that if your breath is fruity smelling, this is a normal sign that you are in ketosis.

This isn't right. This is a closer impression of ketoacidosis, which isn't to be mistaken for supporting ketosis.

You may see a metallic tendency for your mouth when at first beginning keto which is ordinarily fine and not a clarification behind stress, in any case, a fruity smell may show an issue.

CHAPTER FORTEEN

THE GLUCOSE-KETONE RECORD (GKI)

The GKI is another estimation of ketone levels.

It joins your blood glucose and ketone levels into one number, a precise analyzing of your metabolic thriving. Contenders use it to screen their improvement for prosperity and weight objectives.

Experts propose the ketogenic diet for its capacity to chop down blood glucose, which controls diabetes and epilepsy and limits as an undermining advancement treatment. Risky advancement cells feed on glucose. No glucose deduces starving and slaughtering danger cells.

High ketone levels can't perform its responsibility aside from if glucose levels are likewise low. High blood glucose oppositely impacts your success.

CARB CERTIFICATION AND STRESS

Your blood glucose is influenced by hormone apexes and plunges (especially for ladies), healing conditions like diabetes and glandular issues and by your carb assertion and conclusions of uneasiness.

You may need to change your carb far reaching scale to hold your blood glucose down.

Stress triggers cortisol and epinephrine (expand hormones) into spiking your blood glucose for the battle to come or flight. Strategies for controlling weight combine yoga, consideration, interests like planting, drawing, shading and regardless of something as immediate as a long hold the shower.

CHAPTER FIFTEEN

VERY MUCH ARRANGED HEADINGS TO ASSESS YOUR GKI

The condition for deciding the GKI is:

GKI = (Blood Glucose (mg/dL)/18)/Blood Ketones (mmol/L)

1.   Measure your blood glucose a practically identical way you measure your BHB levels on the blood meter (utilizing the right strips).

2.   Divide your glucose number by 18 to change over it to mmol/L. In the event that it's beginning at now in mmol/L, skirt this development.

3.   Divide your glucose number by your ketone level number.

4.   The remaining bit is your GKI number.

GKI Numbers by Objective or Treatment:

A GKI some spot in the extent of 3 and 8 would see you through your weight decline objectives on the ketogenic diet. Here are the broadly perceived GKI estimations as indicated by objectives and conditions/treatment:

•	GKI more than 9: not in ketosis

•	GKI 6-9, low part of ketosis: Significant for weight reduction and impeccable flourishing and weight

•	GKI 3-6, moderate ketosis: The ideal part of ketosis for keeping an eye out for insulin obstruction, type 2 diabetes and heartiness the board

•	GKI of under 3, unusual state of ketosis: Routinely used to address epilepsy and threat treatment. It is attractive to enter this component of ketosis sporadically dependably for sullying repugnance.

CHAPTER SIXTEEN

MUSCLE VERSUS FAT AFTER PHOTOGRAPHS

Alongside ketone levels and your GKI, your muscle to fat extent is another estimation to seek after for your weight lessening advance on keto.

You could either check your muscle to fat extent again utilizing skinfold calipers or a DEXA degree, or measure your progress from photographs.

Continue taking pictures, from the essential photograph to gouge your muscle to fat extent, to no matter what similarly as month to month advance photographs. Subordinate upon your essential estimations and any alteration frameworks you executed to activate ketosis, you would perceive how the ketogenic diet's fat eating up has changed your body structure.

CHAPTER SEVENTEEN

TAPE ESTIMATIONS

A segment of the time, the scale isn't moving yet that doesn't mean you're not getting alive and well.

Your body weight is stunning difficulty to hormonal insecurities, water upkeep and particular fragments, so it's a keen plan to in addition take estimations.

Measure on a practically identical see unavoidably, utilizing a similar evaluating tape and laying it level around your midsection and hips. For your arms, thighs and calves, measure on the amazing side. (I.e., in case you're correct given, measure your correct arm).

Like muscle to fat extent following, tape estimations can be satisfying in demonstrating totally how much muscle to fat extent you've lost.

Scale

The scale is significant in picking your beginning weight. Notwithstanding, in context of the water weight you lose, and in light of how muscle is heavier than fat, the scale isn't as dependable as testing your ketones and the muscle to fat extent and tape estimations when checking your improvement.

MAKING CHANGES ACCORDING TO YOUR KETO DIET

In the wake of following the ketogenic diet satisfactorily long to change your macros as per results, do you feel the need for further adjustments?

For instance, some keto-ers feel so remarkable reasonably and physically that they advance toward getting the chance to be prosperity devotees, and begin to do irregular ketogenic or focused on ketogenic eats less as required.

Some keto-ers also understand how to change their objective setting as shown by their outcomes. Somebody relentlessly shedding 2 pounds seven days changes his or her weight decline goals. Right when a measurement is cultivated, another change breaks past it.

The most outstanding difference in all is to actuate ketosis, or get in reality into it.

CHAPTER EIGHTEEN

THE BEST PROCEDURE TO ADJUST TO ACTUATE KETOSIS

Measure and track everything, from your BMR to your ketone levels and GKI, to get an accurate thought of what you have to change.

Results are exceedingly individualistic: some get into ketosis quick, some don't. To incite ketosis, or move from low-level to facilitate ketosis, utilize any of the going with frameworks:

Use coconut oil in your eating schedule. Coconut oil is half 60% MCTs — medium-chain triglycerides — and contains lauric damaging, which vivifies and continues with ketone generation. Counting coconut oil your eating routine can impel your endogenous ketone creation.

Enlargement your fat insistence. Assurance you're inside the extent of fat you chose above for your keto macros and weight diminishing targets. Pick staggering, standard fats from both plant and creature sources. Avocados, eggs, full fat spread or ghee, reduce chocolate, olive oil. Depleting at any rate 60% of calories from fat lifts your ketone creation.

Try irregular fasting. Fasting some spot in the extent of 8 to 23 hours develops your muscle to fat extent's blend and ketone creation.

Attempt fat fasting, a sort of sporadic fasting moreover called smart mimicking. It mirrors an entire smart in light of the manner in which that your body stays in a fasted state paying little notice to whether you're eating mind blowing fats. This gives you the upsides of fasting (expand in ketone creation) and the ketogenic diet—mind and body filled by ketones.

Point of confinement your carbs. Go as low-carb as you can comprehend how to cripple your glycogen stores. Each individual has varying estimations of carb obstruction expected to actuate ketosis. Yours quality not be what you starting late thought it was. For instance, some accomplish ketosis at 20g of net carbs reliably, while some can accomplish or remain in ketosis at 40g.

Growth your physical improvement. This may work of draining your glycogen stores, raising your ketone age and getting you into ketosis.

Note: It might set aside your body a long chance to conform to utilizing ketones for importance. Amidst this time, it's alright to keep practice at any rate. You may encounter some keto signs which wire torpidity.

Keep up satisfactory protein use. Too little protein and you lose mass and keep the few fragments from your body that can't utilize ketones as a noteworthiness source, similar to parts of your red platelets, kidneys and mind. An unnecessary proportion of protein and you control ketone age. Assurance you gobble up enough protein to support your essential breaking points, in any case not all that much that protein changes into your other glycogen source.

An elegant protein affirmation of 0.55 to 0.77 pounds per body weight incites and deals with ketosis.

Take exogenous ketones. Exogenous ketones give you a touch of MCTs, raise your ketone levels and fat affirmation, moving fat-change and ketone creation. On the off chance that you do convulsive fasting, exogenous ketones enable you to energetic.

Every so often, the separation among progression and agitating is a strong assistance base. In the event that you go facing question among loved ones, disregard it and go past your circle.

Online life has changed into a flourishing framework. Post on Instagram with the advantage hashtag and you can diagram new relationship with individuals crosswise over landmasses, with individuals in precisely a comparative watercraft, with accurately comparable goals, who should consider you responsible for your dedication and be content with you and your movement!

The principal burden is deception can occur. Try to check what you read or hear before considering, acknowledging or sharing anything.

Oblige us in the Ideal Keto Society for a fun, strong party, condition thoughts and to guarantee you're getting affirmations straight about the ketogenic diet.

The giveaways and purposes of constrainment on all things keto fundamentally add to the strategy.

The Ketogenic Diet isn't a "Heap abatement Diet"

The ketogenic diet begins ketosis, a quantifiable condition of handling that can be an outstanding technique to oversee getting progressively thin through fat eating up.

Since it fuses your ingestion, your outcomes will be awesome to you, paying little regard to whether it's a quicker or slower weight decline. The ketogenic diet is a routine used to treat and oversee infection and advance when in doubt wellbeing weight abatement is only a reward. In any case, the constitution of finishing keto still relies on how you execute it.

Endeavor not to surrender if the going has every one of the reserves of being moderate.

Keep up your genius in testing your ketone levels, following your macros and your outcomes. You're getting sound. That is stunning movement!

www.ingramcontent.com/pod-product-compliance
Lightning Source LLC
Chambersburg PA
CBHW051445140726
47987CB00006B/2548